The Student's Guide to Fitness, Nutrition, and Sanity

Table of Contents

Chapter 1. Introduction

Unlock the secret to empowering your mind, body, and spirit with "The Student's Guide to Fitness, Nutrition, and Sanity." This all-encompassing Special Report, designed specifically for students like you, explores the art and science of maintaining a healthy lifestyle while juggling the multifaceted demands of student life. Crafted with love and precision, it offers refreshing insights into fitness, practical and easy-to-follow nutritional guidelines, and proven techniques to retain your sanity during nerve-wracking academic pressures. Let this exciting resource be your compass guiding you towards a balanced, fulfilling life packed full of academic triumphs, personal growth, and utmost vitality. Stay fit, eat right, keep sane, and conquer your student years like a star!

Chapter 2. Understanding the Student Body: Physical Fitness Demystified

Physical fitness is an essential aspect to retaining energy, focus, and overall health, especially for busy students. Its importance can be comprehensively broken down into the following topics.

2.1. Understanding Physical Fitness

Physical fitness goes beyond simply working out at the gym or running for miles. It is defined as a state of health where the body can perform day-to-day activities without fatigue. Two main components define physical fitness: endurance and strength. Cardiovascular endurance is the body's ability to deliver oxygen and nutrients to tissues and remove waste over sustained periods. On the other hand, muscular strength relates to the maximal force a muscle or muscle group can exert during contraction. Both of these are crucial to maintaining optimal health and performance as a student.

2.2. The Importance of Physical Fitness

The benefits of physical fitness extend far beyond a toned physique. Regular physical activity has a profound impact on the body, mind, and academic performance. Physically active students often find improved concentration, memory, and mood, offering an enhanced academic experience. Physical fitness bolsters the immune system, which reduces susceptibility to illness. Moreover, it helps regulate sleep patterns, a critical aspect of student life often disregarded.

2.3. Creating a Fitness Routine

Establishing a fitness routine might seem daunting initially, but it integrates seamlessly into your student life once you get the hang of it. A smart place to start is by determining your fitness goals and breaking them down into achievable tasks. This could be as simple as climbing the stairs to your classes instead of taking the elevator, or walking or biking instead of driving.

Next, identify activities you enjoy; this could be dancing, swimming, team sports, or yoga. The key is to make fitness fun so that it doesn't become a chore. Schedule your workouts like you would any other important activity. It is recommended that students get at least 30 minutes of moderate-intensity physical activity most days of the week, or 150 minutes in total.

2.4. Understanding Nutrition and Fitness

Nutrition and fitness go hand in hand. Proper nutrition fuels your workouts and helps your body recover and build muscle. Oftentimes, busy students make the mistake of prioritizing one over the other. However, physical activity and dietary habits are two sides of the same coin when it comes to health and fitness.

To break it down simply, exercise uses up energy, and food provides the energy required by your body. Consuming a balanced diet ensures that your body gets the essential macro and micronutrients it needs to function optimally.

2.5. Fitness Mistakes to Avoid

While embarking on a fitness journey, it is normal to make mistakes. Awareness of the common pitfalls can help you avoid them and make your fitness journey more effective and enjoyable. Overtraining, not allowing your body to rest and recover, setting unrealistic goals, ignoring nutrition or hydration, and compromising on sleep are some errors students often make.

However, being cognizant about your body's abilities and limitations, prioritizing nutrition and sleep equally as exercise, setting achievable goals, and giving your body ample time to rest, you can avoid most mistakes.

Physical fitness is a lifelong commitment but remember not to let it burden your mind. Instead, let it uplift your body, mind, and spirit. The journey towards achieving physical fitness is as important as the destination. Make the journey enjoyable, and the destination will arrive sooner than you think.

2.6. Embrace the Change

While diving into the world of physical fitness, remember that change is the only constant. Your body will adapt, and so should your exercises. Every few weeks, mix your routine to challenge different muscle groups. Try new activities, vary your exercises, adjust your food habits, or even change your workout times to keep things fresh. This not only helps you stay committed but also ensures you don't hit a plateau in your progress.

Above all else, ensure that your journey towards physical fitness is a process you enjoy and grow through, learning to respect your body's abilities and limits. Strive for progress, not perfection, balancing out your student responsibilities with your health goals. Remember to celebrate your victories, both big and small, as you navigate through this journey towards a stronger, healthier you.

2.7. Conclusion

As a student, striving for physical fitness is one of the most beneficial things you can do for yourself. Not only does it improve your physique and health, but it can also drastically enhance your academic performance and overall wellness. Choose activities that bring you joy, pair exercise with balanced nutrition, listen to your body, and always strive for balance. Make fitness a part of your lifestyle, and you will surely thrive just as brightly outside the classroom as you do inside it.

Chapter 3. Fueling the Brain: Exploring Nutrition for Cognitive Performance

The advent of scientific research into the role of nutrition in cognitive function shows that our dietary choices can significantly influence our academic performance. While we tend to prioritize exercise when thinking about a healthy lifestyle, food – the fuel of our cognitive vehicle – is of undeniable importance.

3.1. Understanding Nutrition: The Brain's Fuel

Your brain, a crucial organ driving your learning, mood, memory, and concentration, consumes a massive amount of your daily energy intake. Although your brain only represents about 2% of your body weight, it consumes approximately 20% of your daily caloric intake. An optimal intake of nutrients helps the brain function efficiently.

Proteins, fats (particularly omega-3 fatty acids), complex carbs, vitamins and minerals — all play significant roles in brain health. Having an optimal balance of these nutrients is essential for fostering brain function and overall mental wellness.

3.2. The Effects of Carbohydrates on Cognitive Function

Carbohydrates, as the primary energy source for the brain, have a central role in cognitive performance. They're your body's main source of glucose – the brain's primary energy substrate. Hence not all carbohydrates are created equal.

Complex carbohydrates, like whole grains, beans, fruits, and vegetables, provide sustained energy for your brain. Conversely, processed carbohydrates or simple sugars provide short-term energy but they cause an energy crash that can impair cognitive function. Opt for carbs with a low glycemic index — foods that cause only a slow rise in blood sugar and insulin levels.

Food	Glycemic Index
Whole Wheat Bread	69
Brown Rice	68
Apple	39
Kidney Beans	24

3.3. Protein's Role in Brain Health

Proteins are composed of building blocks called amino acids. Of the 20 amino acids that proteins provide, nine are essential, meaning our body can't produce them; they must be sourced from our diet. Several of these essential amino acids are critical for brain health. For example, the amino acid tryptophan is a precursor for serotonin, a neurotransmitter essential for mood regulation and fostering a sense of well-being.

Dietary protein is found in foods like fish, meat, poultry, dairy, eggs, legumes, and nuts. It's important to consume an array of these foods to guarantee a diverse intake of all necessary amino acids.

3.4. The Importance of Healthy Fats for Cognitive Performance

Fat forms the majority of your brain and provides insulation for brain cells, optimizing the speed at which information travels.

Omega-3 fatty acids are vital to maintain and improve mental health and cognitive function. They're primary components of neuron cell membranes and are integral for neuronal communication.

DHA, a specific type of Omega-3 fatty acid, is vital for brain health, helping to improve your memory and cognitive function. Foods rich in Omega-3 fatty acids include fatty fish, walnuts, chia seeds, flax seeds, and fortified products like eggs.

Food	Omega-3 fatty acids (g) per Batch
Salmon (cooked, 3 oz.)	1.8
Flaxseeds (ground, 1tbsp)	1.6
Walnuts (14 halves)	2.6
Chia seeds (1 tbsp)	2.5

3.5. The Influence of Vitamins and Minerals on Cognitive Function

For cognitive function, specific vitamins and minerals have higher importance. They play significant roles in maintaining neuronal function, synthesizing neurotransmitters, and regulating homocysteine levels, high levels of which may increase the risk of cognitive decline.

B-vitamins, particularly B6, B9, and B12, are involved in homocysteine metabolism and are connected to cognitive performance. Fruits, vegetables, meat, eggs, and dairy are great sources of these B-vitamins.

Minerals such as iron, zinc, and iodine are critical too. Iron has a pivotal role in oxygen transportation to the brain, supporting cognitive performance. Zinc is crucial for neurotransmitter function and neurons' communication. Iodine is essential for thyroid function, improperly contributing to reduced cognitive function when deficient. Foods rich in these minerals vary from meat, shellfish, seeds, nuts, dairy, to grains and dark chocolate.

Food	Iron (mg)	Zinc (mg)	Iodine (µg)
Beef (cooked, 3 oz.)	2.1	7.0	3.7
Spinach (cooked, 1/2 cup)	3.2	0.8	1.1
Lentils (cooked, 1/2 cup)	3.3	1.3	2.9
Pumpkin seeds (1 ounce)	4.2	2.2	4.8

3.6. Long-Term Dietary Strategy for Brain Health

Planning and following a diet based on these guidelines may seem overwhelming at first, but gradually incorporating these elements into your lifestyle can result in significant improvements in your cognitive performance.

Start with simple, small changes instead of an abrupt dietary overhaul. Include a serving of fruits and vegetables in your meals, opt for whole grains instead of processed cereals, include a source of lean protein in your diet, and avoid sugary beverages and snacks. Slowly introduce omega-3 rich foods and ensure you're consuming adequate vitamins and minerals.

Remember to keep your food choices diverse - different foods come with varying sets of vital nutrients. As your dietary habits begin to change, you could see noticeable improvements in your concentration, memory, and overall cognitive performance.

Achieving a balanced diet promotes not just cognitive performance but also physical health, mood, and overall quality of life. Empower your brain by feeding it the right fuel, and it will propel your academic performance to new altitudes. Being a student doesn't mean health takes a back seat, it means it should take the front seat to support your academic success. So, choose wisely; your brain and body will thank you.

In the next chapter, we will explore keeping your body moving with effective fitness techniques — the perfect complement to a brain-boosting diet — and provide you the ultimate mind-body curriculum.

Chapter 4. The Resilient Mind: Strategies for Managing Academic Stress

Studying can be a stressful process. As a student, you're often asked to balance a high-powered academic workload with personal life, extracurricular activities, and physical wellness. This chapter will introduce several strategies to help manage academic stress effectively and promote resilience, divided into various subsections: understanding stress, building a resilience mindset, prioritizing self-care, and employing stress management techniques.

4.1. Understanding Stress

First, it's essential to understand what stress is. Stress is your body's natural response to excessive pressure or challenges, often leading to a sense of overwhelm or inability to cope. When faced with a stressful situation, your body releases hormones like adrenaline and cortisol, causing physical changes, such as a faster heartbeat, heightened senses, and increased alertness.

But not all stress is damaging. There's eustress, or positive stress, like the adrenaline rush before a presentation. This can motivate you, boost your performance, and even enhance learning. However, chronic or excessive stress, known as distress, can negatively impact your body and mind, hindering academic performance.

4.2. Building a Resilience Mindset

Resilience refers to your ability to bounce back from difficulties or adapt to change. A resilient mindset is essential in managing academic stress effectively. Here's how to cultivate one:

1. Develop a Growth Mindset: Embrace challenges as opportunities to learn. Rather than focusing on failures, interpret them as valuable feedback that helps you evolve.

2. Practice Mindfulness: A centered and present mind is more resilient. Mindfulness meditation can help enhance focus, clarity, and emotional intelligence.

3. Cultivate Optimism: Learn to focus on the positive without ignoring the negative. An optimistic attitude can make adversity more manageable.

4. Build Resourcefulness: Learn how to find quick and clever solutions to your problems. This includes time management, studying techniques, and problem-solving skills.

4.3. Prioritizing Self-Care

Self-care involves activities and practices we engage in regularly to reduce stress and maintain and enhance our short- and long-term health and well-being. Here are some self-care measures:

1. Physical Exercise: Regular activity helps decrease stress hormones and promotes the release of feel-good hormones like serotonin and endorphins. Aim for moderate exercise like walking, cycling, or yoga for about 30 minutes a day.

2. Balanced Diet: Consuming a balanced diet ensures that your body and brain get the necessary nutrients to function properly.

3. Adequate Sleep: Sleep is crucial for cognitive functions. It not only consolidates memory but also aids in problem-solving and creativity.

4. Social Interactions: Spending quality time with people who enrich your life can provide emotional support and unwind from academic pressures.

4.4. Employing Stress Management Techniques

Effective stress management can drastically improve your quality of life and academic performance. Here are some strategies:

1. Breathing Techniques: A simple deep-breathing exercise can instantly lower stress levels by slowing the heart rate and lowering blood pressure.

2. Progressive Muscle Relaxation (PMR): Tense and then relax each muscle group, starting from your toes and moving up to your head. It promotes physical relaxation and mental calmness.

3. Cognitive Behavioral Therapy (CBT) Techniques: CBT methods, such as cognitive reframing, can help you change detrimental thinking patterns into more constructive ones.

4. Time Management Techniques: Techniques like the Pomodoro method (25 minutes of concentrated work followed by a 5-minute break) can boost productivity.

By understanding stress, building resilience, prioritizing self-care, and employing stress management techniques, you can navigate the whirlwind of academic life calmly and effectively. Remember, it's about progress, not perfection. Learning to manage stress is a journey, not a destination.

Chapter 5. Daily Routines to Boost Your Energy and Mood

Understanding your body's internal clock, or circadian rhythm, can help you create daily routines that naturally enhance your energy and uplift your mood. In this chapter, we'll guide you through how to develop your energy-boosting routine that synchronizes with your body's natural rhythm, maximizing your productivity and well-being.

5.1. Understanding Your Circadian Rhythm

The circadian rhythm is a natural, internal process that regulates the sleep-wake cycle. It repeats roughly every 24 hours and affects not just our sleep, but also our body temperature, hormone levels, and mood. This biological clock is influenced by environmental cues, like sunlight and temperature, but keeping regular hours greatly helps our bodies establish a healthy rhythm.

Understanding your circidian rhythm can have many benefits. By following a routine that works in sync with your body's natural tendencies, you have an opportunity to enjoy energized days and restful nights.

5.2. The Power of Good Morning Routines

How you start your day sets the tone for the rest of it. A solid morning routine helps signal to your body that it's time to awaken and get moving, which in turn can help you feel more awake and energized.

1. Begin the day with a glass of lemon water. This helps kickstart your metabolism and gently wake your body after a night of rest.

2. Engage in a physical activity that suits you. This could be a brisk walk, yoga stretches, or a more intense workout. Exercise in the morning releases endorphins that can enhance your mood and energy levels.

3. Include meditative practices such as breathing exercises, yoga, or mindfulness meditation. These activities can help calm your mind and prepare you to handle the challenges of the day ahead.

4. Have a nutrient-rich breakfast. Incorporate high-fiber cereals, fruits, and protein-rich foods like eggs or Greek yogurt to fuel your body for the day.

5.3. Mental Health and Daily Routine

Following a healthy daily routine can promote better mental health. It provides tasks to focus on, simplicity to understand, and visible progress, all of which can reduce feelings of anxiety.

1. Make time in your daily routine for recreational activities, hobbies, or anything that brings you joy.

2. Incorporate short breaks throughout the day for mindfulness meditation or deep breathing techniques to reduce stress.

3. Schedule social activities. Engaging with friends and family can be a major mood booster, whether through phone calls, online meetings, or face-to-face get-togethers.

4. Get plenty of sleep. Aim for seven to nine hours each night.

5.4. Incorporating Healthy Eating Habits into Your Daily Routine

A balanced diet is crucial in ensuring high energy levels and a stable mood. Here are some tips for incorporating healthy eating habits:

1. Start with a balanced breakfast packed with protein, fiber and a bit of healthy fat to ward off hunger and keep you energized.

2. Plan your meals and snacks in advance to avoid unhealthy, last-minute choices.

3. Stay hydrated. Drinking plenty of water throughout the day can boost your metabolism and help you stay alert.

5.5. The Impact of Sleep on Energy and Mood

Getting a good night's rest is essential for overall vitality. Inadequate sleep can lead to feelings of lethargy and irritability. Here are some ways to encourage quality sleep:

1. Maintain a consistent sleep schedule. Going to bed and waking up at the same time each day can help regulate your body's internal clock and could help you sleep better.

2. Create a pre-sleep routine. Engaging in relaxing activities like reading or taking a hot bath can signal to your body that it's time to sleep.

3. Keep your sleep environment peaceful, dark, and at a comfortable temperature.

As you build energy-enhancing, mood-boosting routines, remember to be flexible. Your routines should assist you, not make you feel excessively restricted. Be patient, and allow yourself to gradually adjust to new routines. Before long, you'll enjoy the renewed vigor and positive outlook that come with them.

Chapter 6. Building Healthy Habits: A Guide for the Busy Student

As a student, maintaining healthy habits may often be pushed to the end of your long to-do list. Yet, incorporating these critical routines into your daily life will not only enhance your academic performance but also boost your overall wellbeing.

6.1. Understanding the Value of Healthy Habits

A habit is a routine behavior that gets repeated subconsciously. When you cultivate good habits, you create a streamlined daily routine that not only saves your mind from the constant negotiations about what to do next but also leads to significant health benefits.

Creating healthy habits is like an investment that pays lifelong dividends. These routines guard your psychological, physical, and emotional health, giving you the energy and mental strength to tackle academic and personal challenges.

6.2. Identifying Key Healthy Habits

There is no one-size-fits-all approach when it comes to creating healthy habits. What works for your roommate might not work for you. However, some fundamental habits generally contribute to good health for students universally:

- Regular exercise
- Balanced nutrition

- Adequate sleep

- Stress management techniques

- Regular health check-ups

These are broad categories, each requiring their comprehensive guide. However, the succeeding sections will provide practical measures to implement these habits in your routine.

6.3. Incorporating Regular Exercise into Your Routine

Exercise offers numerous benefits, from enhancing your mood and energy levels to improving your cognitive function. While it's common for students to skip workouts due to their hectic schedules, regular exercise can make a significant impact on your overall wellbeing.

Keep in mind that exercise doesn't necessarily mean intense gym workouts. Even simple activities like walking to class instead of taking a bus or doing a 15-min yoga routine can significantly contribute to your physical wellness. Here are some strategies:

- Schedule your workouts just like your study or class time, making them non-negotiable.

- Experiment with different forms of exercise until you find one you enjoy. It could be dancing, running, swimming, or biking.

- Take advantage of fitness classes or athletic facilities available at your university.

6.4. Maintaining a Balanced Diet

Nutrition plays a vital role in maintaining your energy levels, concentration, and overall health. While it may be tempting to rely on takeouts or instant meals, including whole foods in your diet can make a significant difference in how you feel and function.

Following are some strategies:

- Plan your meals and snacks ahead of time to prevent reaching for unhealthy options when you're busy or stressed.

- Include a variety of fruits, vegetables, lean proteins, and whole grains in your diet.

- Stay hydrated by drinking ample water throughout the day.

- Limit your intake of sugar and caffeine, which can lead to energy crashes later in the day.

6.5. Ensuring Adequate Sleep

Sleep often becomes a luxury for many students, especially during exam periods. However, sleep is critical for cognitive functions like memory consolidation, creativity, and problem-solving.

Here are some practical steps to ensure a good night's rest:

- Establish a regular sleep schedule, aiming for 7-9 hours of sleep every night.

- Create a relaxing pre-sleep routine, like reading or meditating, to prepare your body for rest.

- Limit your exposure to electronic devices at least an hour before bed.

6.6. Managing Stress Efficiently

The demanding nature of student life can lead to chronic stress, taking a significant toll on your mind and body.

Here are several ways to manage stress:

- Practice mindfulness or meditation. Even a few minutes of daily meditation can help improve your mental health.

- Reach out to friends, family, or a trusted counselor when feeling overwhelmed.

- Indulge in creative activities, hobbies, or anything that brings you joy and relaxation.

6.7. Prioritizing Regular Health Check-ups

While students often neglect this part, regular health check-ups are crucial to early detect any potential health issues.

- Utilize the health services provided by your university or local healthcare provider.

- Keep track of annual physicals, dental check-ups, and eye exams to ensure a holistic approach to health.

6.8. Cultivating Habits: Becoming a Better You

Though incorporating healthy habits can seem challenging at first, regular practice can make them second nature. Remember, it's not about major lifestyle overhauls but small, regular actions that gradually lead towards a healthier lifestyle.

Take one step at a time. Focus on one habit you want to incorporate into your life and stick with it until it becomes natural. Reward yourself when you meet your goals, but be easy on yourself if you slip up. With consistency and patience, you can successfully build a more balanced and nourishing life, ensuring not only your academic success but your overall wellbeing as a student.

Chapter 7. Eating on a Budget: Healthy, Affordable Choices

Eating healthily on a budget can seem like a daunting challenge, especially for students who may face the pressures of time, convenience and inexpensive fast food options. However, it is entirely possible to eat well without overspending. Remember that when you make an investment into your nutrition, you are investing in your health and long-term wellbeing. With strategic planning, savvy shopping, and the right approach to meals and snacks, it becomes easier to feed your body nutritious food without breaking the bank.

7.1. Pantry Essentials

One secret to affordable, healthy eating is a well-stocked pantry. You can save money by choosing versatile, shelf-stable items. The list below outlines budget-friendly staples you can always rely on:

- Whole grains: Rice, oats, whole grain pasta, quinoa, and whole grain bread.

- Canned goods: Canned beans, tomatoes, corn, and tuna.

- Nuts and Seeds: Almonds, peanuts, chia seeds, flaxseeds, etc.

- Dried or canned fruits: Raisins, apricots, cranberries, pineapple, etc.

- Spices and seasonings: Salt, pepper, garlic powder, oregano, cinnamon, etc.

- Oils and Vinegars: Olive oil, canola oil, vinegar, etc.

- Other staples: Nut butter, honey, dark chocolate, granola.

7.2. Savvy Shopping Techniques

Buy in Bulk: Purchasing ingredients in bulk is a cost-effective solution for those foods you frequently consume. Grains like rice, oats, lentils, and beans are usually cheaper when bought in large quantities.

Go Seasonal: Fruits and vegetables are less expensive (and more flavorful!) when they are in season. Also, try to purchase locally to support smaller businesses and save on transportation costs.

Use Sales and Discounts: Keep an eye out for sales and discounts at your local grocery store. Meal planning around sales items can save lots of money in the long run.

Freeze Leftovers: Food waste is also money waste. Freezing leftovers or excess produce will save you money and make cooking more convenient.

7.3. Meal Planning

Meal planning is key to affordable, healthy eating. Plan your meals around the ingredients you already have, then shop for the remaining items needed. Always keep the plan flexible and experiment with different recipes. Investing some time in planning your meals reduces the temptation for takeout and unnecessary purchases.

7.4. Preparing Nutritious, Budget-Friendly Meals

Below are some meal ideas that incorporate the tips mentioned above:

Breakfast: Overnight oats with canned fruits and nuts/seeds. **Lunch**: Whole grain pasta with canned tomatoes, tunas, olives and herbs. **Dinner**: Brown rice, beans, and a vegetable stir-fry. **Snack**: A piece of seasonal fruit, a handful of nuts, or a slice of whole grain bread with nut butter.

Preparing these meals not only saves money, but also ensures a balanced diet.

7.5. Budget Doesn't Mean Boring

Remember, sticking to a budget doesn't mean sacrificing taste or meal variety. Use spices, herbs, and low-cost ingredients like garlic and onions to flavor your foods. And explore different cuisines for inspiration; many global foods are based on inexpensive, whole-food ingredients.

Eating on a budget may feel like a challenge initially. But with awareness, planning, and practice, it can become a sustainable, enjoyable habit. It's truly an investment in good nutrition and your overall well-being. With these guidelines, you're ready to embark on the journey of healthy, affordable eating. Who knew students could be master chefs on a shoestring budget? You're writing the next chapter in your journey toward fitness, nutrition, and sanity. Happy cooking!

Chapter 8. Hitting the Gym: A Beginner's Guide to Effective Workout

Having decided to kickstart a new fitness routine is no less than an accomplishment itself. However, the world of the gymnasium, with its plethora of machines, weights, and routines, can often feel bewildering to the uninitiated. This chapter aims to shine a light on the essentials that may help you navigate the gym confidently, effectively, and potentially injury-free.

8.1. Choosing Your Gym

Selecting the right gym is first and foremost. Consider factors like proximity, cost, cleanliness, and the range of facilities. Many gyms offer trial periods or day passes - take advantage of this before committing to a long-term contract. It's essential that you feel comfortable in the physical space and, to an extent, align with the gym's overall vibe and ethos.

8.2. Starting with a Plan

Approaching the gym without a plan can lead to unproductive sessions. Outline a broad arrangement of your workout structure, complete with goals. This might be a balance of cardio and strength training, weight loss, muscle building or improving general fitness. Don't be disheartened if progress seems slow - fitness is not a one-size-fits-all, and achieving goals takes time.

8.3. The Importance of a Warm-Up

The benefits of a proper warm-up cannot be stressed enough. Warming up prepares your body for a workout, getting the blood flowing to your muscles and making them more pliable and less prone to injuries. At least 5-10 minutes of dynamic movements, like brisk walking or light jogging, can suffice as an effective warm-up.

8.4. Introduction to Cardio

Most gyms offer a variety of cardio machines - treadmills, stationary bikes, ellipticals, stair climbers, and rowing machines. These devices are perfect for beginners, offering an excellent way to get your heart rate up. Start with short segments - 10 to 20 minutes, gradually increasing the duration as your fitness level improves.

8.5. Strength Training Basics

Strength training is an integral part of any exercise routine that helps in muscular development and endurance. Most people jump onto machines without realizing that bodyweight exercises like push-ups, squats, lunges, and pull-ups are also effective. When moving to weights, begin with small ones, slowly increasing the amount as strength grows.

8.6. Navigating Workout Machines

The variety of workout machines in a gym can often be intimidating. Start with the simple ones - leg press, chest press, seated row, lat pulldown, and shoulder press. Remember, machines often have instructional diagrams attached. When in doubt, it's good to ask a fitness professional for some assistance.

8.7. Importance of Correct Form

The right form is paramount when exercising. It ensures that the right muscles are engaged in the movement, and significantly reduces the risk of injury. Don't let ego be your guide - it's always better to lift lighter weights correctly than heavier weights incorrectly.

8.8. Breathing: The Understated Hero

Correct breathing is essential, often understated component of a beneficial workout. As a general rule, exhale during the exertion part of an exercise (like lifting or pushing) and inhale during the less strenuous part (like lowering or relaxing).

8.9. Taking Rest Periods

Rest is integral - it's your body's time to recuperate and grow stronger. Between sets, a rest duration of 30-90 secs is suggested. Also, ensuring that you get enough sleep each night gets you ready for the next day's workout.

8.10. The Cool-Down Phase

Just as you warm up, you should cool down after a workout. It helps in gradually returning your heart rate and blood pressure to their resting states. Stretching exercises are a great way to cool down and promote flexibility at the same time.

8.11. Listening to Your Body

Last but not least, listen to your body. If something hurts or doesn't feel right, stop. Take a break when you're ill. Be kind to your body and respect the signals it sends you; it's the only one you have.

Remember, embarking on a journey of fitness is a commitment of time and patience. With informed choices, dedicated efforts, and consistency, the transformation you aspire for is attainable. Don't strain yourself on the very first day; start slowly and build steadily. Welcome to the gym!

Chapter 9. Rest and Recovery: The Forgotten Aspect of Fitness

Your dedication to fitness must be balanced by understanding its less-discussed counterpart - rest and recovery. Herein lies the key to effective and sustainable physical health. As much as we hear about the importance of working out, the role of rest and recovery time in achieving fitness goals is just as critical.

9.1. Understanding the Importance of Rest and Recovery

The human body operates like a finely tuned machine, with each part playing a vital role. When you exercise, your body's muscles experience a form of stress. They break down and cause microscopic damage. This is entirely normal and a necessary precursor to muscle regeneration and growth.

But to rebuild, your body needs to experience recovery. Think of it as a construction project. The demolition phase is akin to a workout when your body experiences stress and breakage. The rebuilding or recovery phase is when repair occurs. Fuelled by the right nutrients and adequate rest, your muscles heal and grow stronger, preparing you for your next workout.

9.2. The Difference Between Rest and Recovery

Despite the terms being used interchangeably, rest and recovery are not the same. Properly distinguishing between them can help you maximize your fitness outcomes.

Rest refers to the periods of relaxation or sleep that you incorporate into your daily schedule. It's often assessed by the amount of sleep you get every night, but can also include periods of calm during the day.

Recovery, on the other hand, is a more encompassing term. It refers to techniques and actions, like post-workout nutrition, stretching, and stress management, that help your body recuperate after physical activity and maintain a balanced state of health over time.

9.3. The Art of Active Rest

Rest needn't mean complete inactivity. Engaging in low-intensity activities or 'active rest' allows your body to recuperate while remaining moderately active. Activities like light swimming, cycling, or yoga can increase blood flow, hasten muscle recovery, and lift your mood. Determining the right blend of active and passive rest is a matter of personal context and fitness levels.

9.4. Importance of Sleep

Sleep is a crucial component of rest. During sleep, your body goes into an intense recovery mode. Growth hormone, one of the primary agents of muscle repair and recovery, is released during the deep stages of sleep.

Irregular or inadequate sleep patterns can rob you of these restorative periods, slowing muscle recovery, and compromising your immune system. Aim for 7-9 hours of sleep per night and consider short power naps if your schedule permits during the day.

9.5. Post-Workout Nutrition

When it comes to recovery, your post-exercise meal is an absolute game-changer. Proper nourishment allows your body to rebuild glycogen stores and repair damaged muscles.

A balance of carbs and protein within a window of about 45 minutes post-workout is typically recommended. Healthy examples include grilled chicken with brown rice and vegetables, a protein shake with banana, or low-fat Greek yogurt with fresh berries.

9.6. Hydration Matters

Staying hydrated is crucial for recovery. Water regulates body temperature, helps with digestion, and aids nutrient absorption – all key to recovery. Dehydration can lead to muscle cramps and fatigue, lowering your performance levels. Aim for half of your body weight (in pounds) in ounces of water each day and increase the intake around your workouts.

9.7. Prioritizing Stretch and Recovery Workouts

Often sidelined in fitness routines, stretching and recovery workouts are vital for preventing injuries and boosting flexibility. Practices like yoga or Pilates can improve your muscle potential and offer mental health benefits.

9.8. Say Yes to Massages

Massages or self-myofascial release, using tools like foam rollers, can improve circulation, aid in removing toxins, and speed up recovery time. They can also help reduce muscle soreness after a hard workout.

9.9. Managing Stress

Stress can drain your body and compromise your recovery capacity. Incorporating stress-busting techniques such as meditation, deep-breathing or gentle yoga can significantly improve your recovery potential.

9.10. Listen to Your Body

Lastly, always listen to your body. It knows when it needs rest. Chronic fatigue, changes in sleep patterns, or decreased performance could signal that your body needs more recovery time.

Investing time and efforts into recovery can significantly elevate your fitness levels and overall health. By paying attention to both your workouts and your rest and recovery, you're setting the foundations of a holistic fitness approach that will sustain you throughout your student years and beyond. Your body and mind will thank you.

Chapter 10. The Social Aspect of Wellness: Connections, Community, and Mental Health

Understanding the integral role that our relationships and social interactions play in our overall wellness is a significant part of maintaining balanced and vibrant health – both physically and mentally. This becomes even more pertinent when considered within the context of student life, where interactions, networks, and societies forge significant aspects of our academic experience.

10.1. Identifying your Social Needs

While each person has unique social needs, there are common elements that form our basic requirements. These can range from the need for companionship and shared experiences to emotional support, intellectual stimulation, and the necessity to both give and receive assistance in times of crisis or difficulty.

As a student, identifying your social needs can be a complex process. You're continuously dealing with a melting pot of cultures, ideas, and personalities, which can sometimes be overwhelming. However, recognizing what you need from social interactions to thrive emotionally and intellectually is essential. Remember, it's not about fitting into a specific social box; it's about satisfying your holistic wellness needs.

Conduct self-reflection exercises and introspections often to understand better what you seek from social connections. Understand your comfort zones, identify the people and interactions draining your energy, and distinguish the ones that inspire and uplift you.

10.2. Building a Supportive Network

Creating a supportive network doesn't happen overnight. It's an ongoing process based on mutual respect and shared interests. Your environment as a student provides countless opportunities to meet a diverse range of people, each with their unique perspectives. Here are some strategies to build a supportive social network:

1. Seek out like-minded individuals: Join clubs, organizations, or anything that aligns with your hobbies, passions, and interests. By doing this, you're likely to meet individuals who you share common ground with, making it easier to form meaningful connections.

2. Communicate effectively: Be open, transparent, and accepting in your conversations. Remember that everyone has their own unique story and experiences, which can lead to enriching discussions and mutual understanding.

3. Be respectful and compassionate: Understand that each individual is fighting their own battles. Mutual respect and empathy can go a long way in fostering strong relations.

4. Help and accept help: Community-building is not just about asking for help, but also about lending a helping hand when one can. This interaction creates a circle of shared trust and reciprocity, strengthening your network in the process.

10.3. Dealing with Loneliness and Isolation

Being away from home or in a new environment can often lead to feelings of loneliness and isolation. It's common for students to undergo periods of solitude, whether it's due to homesickness or grappling with the new academically demanding environment.

Here are some effective strategies for dealing with these feelings:

1. Get involved: Involve yourself in various campus activities or pursue a new hobby or interest, this helps form connections and keeps loneliness at bay.

2. Seek support: Don't hesitate to use available resources, such as counseling services provided by your school. They are equipped to handle exactly these scenarios and can provide you with useful strategies and coping mechanisms.

3. Engage in self-care: Loneliness can sometimes be overwhelming, and it's easy to forget to take care of yourself. Establish a routine that includes exercise, good nutrition, and activities you find relaxing or enjoyable.

10.4. Embracing Diversity

The modern-day student environment is a melting pot of cultures, religions, and ethnicities. Embracing diversity enriches your worldview, broadens your thinking, and can also help inculcate valuable skills like adaptability and tolerance.

Here are some ways to embrace diversity:

1. Educate yourself: Understand and learn about different cultures, religions, and beliefs. This knowledge aids tolerance and mutual respect.

2. Engage in open conversations: Discussion promotes understanding. Do not shy away from asking questions or sharing your own experiences and viewpoints, as long as it's done respectfully.

3. Take part in multicultural events: Many university campuses organize multicultural events and festivals. Participating in these

events is an enriching experience and brilliant way to acknowledge and appreciate diversity.

10.5. Concluding Thoughts

The social aspect of our wellness is a fundamental part of our overall health. As a student, it becomes crucial to understand this interconnected relationship, truly acknowledging the impact of our social interactions on our mental and physical health.

The strategies mentioned above offer a comprehensive guide to nurture the social aspect of your wellness, dealing proactively with related challenges. Remember, the ultimate goal is to establish a balance between your academic requirements, personal needs, and social commitments in such a way that promotes overall wellness and growth.

Keeping this balance is a journey that will see changes and require adjustments along the way but ensuring that it's given the importance it deserves will undoubtedly result in a fulfilling, healthy, and successful student life.

Chapter 11. Long-term Fitness: Sustainability in Your Health Journey

Healthy living is not just about making dramatic changes for short-term results; it's about incorporating lasting changes into your routine for long-term sustainability. For students, surviving the chaos of academic life while remaining physically fit might seem daunting. However, the secret lies in making manageable yet effective adjustments to your daily routine.

11.1. Understanding Fitness Sustainability

Fitness is a lifelong commitment, not a seasonal endeavor. It's about developing healthy habits that you can maintain in the long term. In the context of a student's life, sustainability means integrating fitness habits that are feasible within their academic schedule, budget, and personal preferences. To achieve a sustainably fit lifestyle, understanding and assimilating the principles of consistency, balance, and adaptability is crucial.

1. Consistency: The key to long-term fitness is not the intensity of your workout but regularity. Regular physical activity brings gradual improvement, which is more beneficial and sustainable than quick, dramatic changes brought by intense yet sporadic workouts.

2. Balance: Striking a balance between different types of exercises and recovery is essential. Include a mix of cardio, strength training, and flexibility exercises in your routine. Also, do not overlook the importance of rest days for recovery.

3. Adaptability: University life often involves changes in schedules, circumstances, or locations. The ability to adapt your fitness regimen as per situational constraints is essential for sustainability.

11.2. Building A Consistent Workout Routine

A major challenge students face in maintaining fitness is creating a consistent exercise routine. Here's how you can maintain consistency despite a hectic schedule.

1. Establish a routine: Design an exercise schedule that fits easily into your daily routine. It could be a morning jog, an evening yoga class, or performing bodyweight exercises in your dorm room.

2. Set realistic goals: Unrealistic goals can quickly lead to demotivation. Start with small, achievable objectives that can gradually be increased over time.

3. Make it enjoyable: The more you enjoy your workout, the more likely you'll stay consistent. Choose activities that you find enjoyable whether it's dancing, hiking, swimming, or team sports.

11.3. Balancing Activities for Optimal Health

Balance is crucial in a fitness regimen. Too much of the same exercise can cause repetitive strain injuries and won't work your body in a balanced manner.

1. Mix cardio and strength: Cardiovascular activities improve your heart health while strength training builds muscles and bones. A mix of both ensures overall health benefits.

2. Incorporate flexibility and balance exercises: These exercises improve body functions, prevent injury, and enhance physical performance. Activities such as yoga and Pilates provide combined benefits of flexibility, strength, and balance.

3. Include rest days: Contrary to popular belief, rest days are vital in a fitness regime. Rest aids recovery, promotes muscle growth, and prevents injuries.

11.4. Adapting Your Fitness Routine

Being flexible and adaptable with your fitness routine is crucial for maintaining long-term habits, especially as a student.

1. Adjusting for academic demands: During more demanding academic periods, such as exam weeks, you can adjust your routine. You might shorten your workouts or switch to lower intensity activities.

2. Workout during travel: Staying active while traveling, perhaps for exchange programs or internships, can be challenging. Pack portable exercise equipment, like resistance bands, or use bodyweight workout routines that can be done anywhere.

3. Adapting to injuries: If you're injured and cannot follow your regular exercise routine, adapt to a regime that allows comfortable movements. Consult a healthcare professional for a suitable workout plan during recovery.

11.5. Turning Fitness into a Lifelong Habit

Consistency, balance, and adaptability are the pillars of turning fitness into a lifelong habit. Additionally, adopting the mindset of 'fitness as a lifestyle' rather than 'fitness as a chore' can significantly improve the sustainability of your fitness regime.

Maintaining a sustainably fit lifestyle amidst the dynamic demands of student life may seem challenging. However, with the right approach and mindset, prioritizing your health can pave the way to academic success. By understanding the principles of fitness sustainability, you're not just committing to a fitter you for a few semesters, but for life.